# CARNIVORE DIET COOKBOOK FOR BEGINNERS

**The Complete And Easy Recipes That Guild Beginners To Nourishing The Primal Palate**

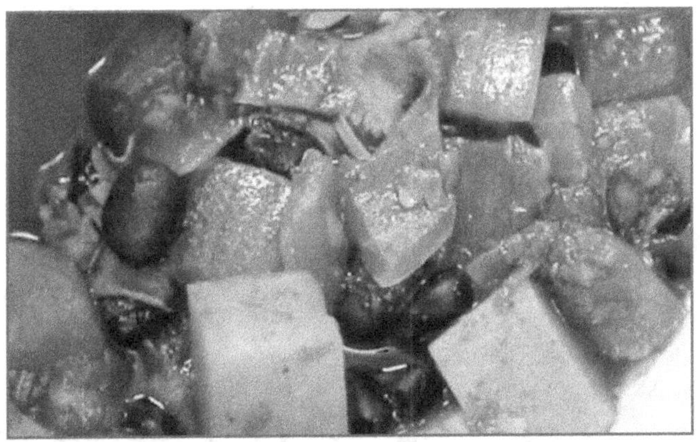

# Reina W. Edmonds

# Copyright



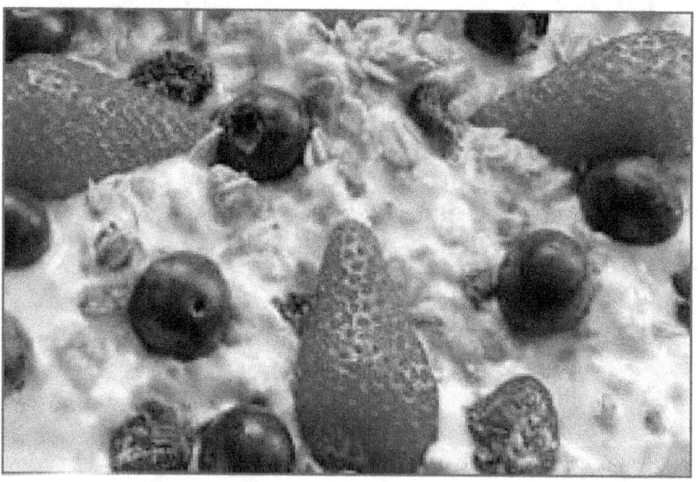

# TABLE OF CONTENT

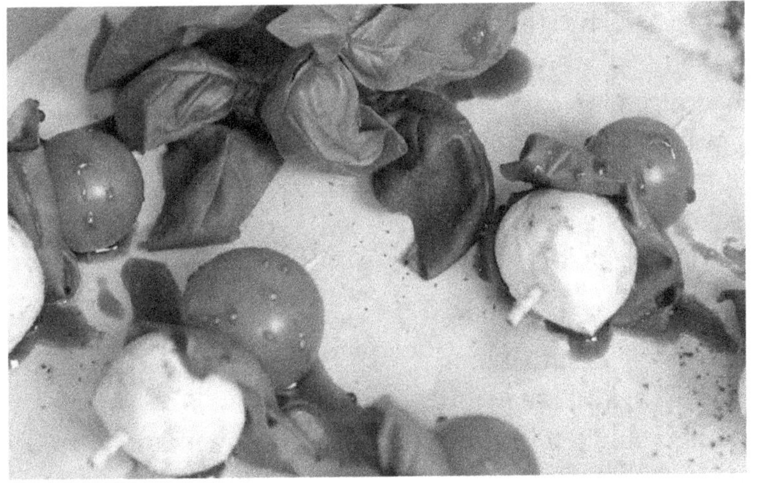

# INTRODUCTION

Fitness enthusiast Sarah decided to follow the Carnivore Diet to improve her energy and overall health. As a novice, she had to figure out how to make tasty, filling meals while adhering to the regimen. She was fortunate enough to come upon the "Carnivore Delights Cookbook for Beginners."

Motivated by the thoughtful preface of the cookbook, Sarah explored the realm of meat-based staples, becoming an expert in both meat selection and cooking methods. She was able to organize her daily intake and maintain a balanced approach to the carnivorous lifestyle thanks to the thorough meal planning part.

Her daily regimen followed the breakfast dishes, including creative lamb breakfast chops, bacon variants, and steak and eggs. Sarah had steak patties, grilled chicken salads, and healthy prawn and avocado dishes for lunch. Savory ribeye steaks, exotic fish fillets, and herb-crusted lamb chops turned dinner into a gourmet excursion.

The cookbook's easy-to-make snacks, such as the enticing parmesan crisps, cheese rolls, and beef jerky, easily satiated snack cravings. Sarah's Carnivore Diet adventure evolved into a culinary adventure and a health shift because of the knowledgeable advice and delicious dishes in her go-to cookbook. Her successful transition to a predatory lifestyle was demonstrated by her increased energy and vitality, which led her to become an enthusiastic supporter of this novel dietary strategy.

## *The Carnivore Diet: What Is It?*

A dietary strategy known as the "Carnivore Diet" centers on consuming just meat and other animal items exclusively. It is a drastic divergence from standard dietary recommendations in that it excludes any plant-based foods, such as grains, fruits, and vegetables. Proponents stress the nutritional value of animal products and contend that our predecessors survived on a diet comparable to theirs. To maximize health and well-being, the Carnivore Diet usually promotes the intake of red meat, poultry, fish, and other goods originating from animals.

## *Advantages of a Carnivorous Diet*

The possible health advantages of the Carnivore Diet are highly regarded. Advocates claim that it can result in greater energy, better mental clarity, and weight reduction. Furthermore, some people report decreased inflammation and relief from certain medical illnesses including autoimmune diseases. The diet's focus on animal items high in nutrients supplies vital vitamins and minerals that promote general wellness. Individual reactions may differ, and it's important to remember that scientific agreement on the safety and long-term implications of the carnivore diet is still developing.

## *Welcome and Overview*

Starting a Carnivore Diet takes thorough preparation and comprehension. Beginning with a gradual shift allows the body to adjust to the altered nutritional makeup. Removing plant-based diets and carbs may cause some early difficulties, including the "keto flu." Learning about appropriate meat choices, cooking methods, and quantity management is crucial. It's also a good idea to speak with a healthcare provider before beginning the Carnivore Diet to be sure it fits with your particular health objectives and concerns. The groundwork for an enjoyable and long-lasting voyage into the realm of carnivorous eating is laid during this initial phase.

# CHAPTER 1
# Comprehending Carnivorous Foods

## *1.1 Meat Choosing Guide*

A key to successfully implementing the Carnivore Diet is selecting the appropriate meats. People may use the Meat Selection Guide as a compass to help them navigate the complex world of animal products. To maintain optimal nutritional content, emphasis is put on choosing high-quality meats, ideally those grown on pasture or grass. Because of their high protein and fat content, varieties such as beef, lamb, chicken, and fatty fish are advised. By helping to differentiate between lean and fatty cuts, the guide helps practitioners match their meat selections to their nutritional needs and dietary preferences. A well-rounded and fulfilling carnivorous diet plan may be made by persons who are knowledgeable about the subtleties of meat choosing.

## 1.2 Preparing Food Methods

The use of carnivore cooking methods is essential for enhancing the flavor and texture of food without sacrificing its nutritious value. Roasting, grilling, searing, and slow cooking are some of the popular ways to prepare meats. A Carnivore Diet Cookbook's section on cooking techniques explores how to enhance flavors without sacrificing the diet's core tenets. It looks at enhancing meals with animal fats, spices, and herbs. Furthermore, emphasis is placed on cooking temperatures and timings to guarantee food safety while preserving preferred textures and flavors. When these methods are mastered, carnivore staples become delectable gourmet creations, elevating the diet from a dietary decision to a culinary journey.

## 1.3 Vital Components

A Carnivore Diet includes necessary elements that support the nutritional objectives of the diet in addition to its main concentration on meats. Rich in vitamins and minerals, organ meats like kidney and liver add to a well-rounded nutritional profile. Tallow and lard are examples of animal fats that are useful as cooking oils and as sources of good fats. Another essential is eggs, which may be used to make a wide range of foods. The section on Essential Ingredients guides individuals on how to incorporate these ingredients into their diets, therefore guaranteeing a holistic approach to nutrition. Through the use of this variety of carnivore-friendly foods, practitioners may optimize the nutritional advantages and gastronomic variety of their carnivorous way of life.

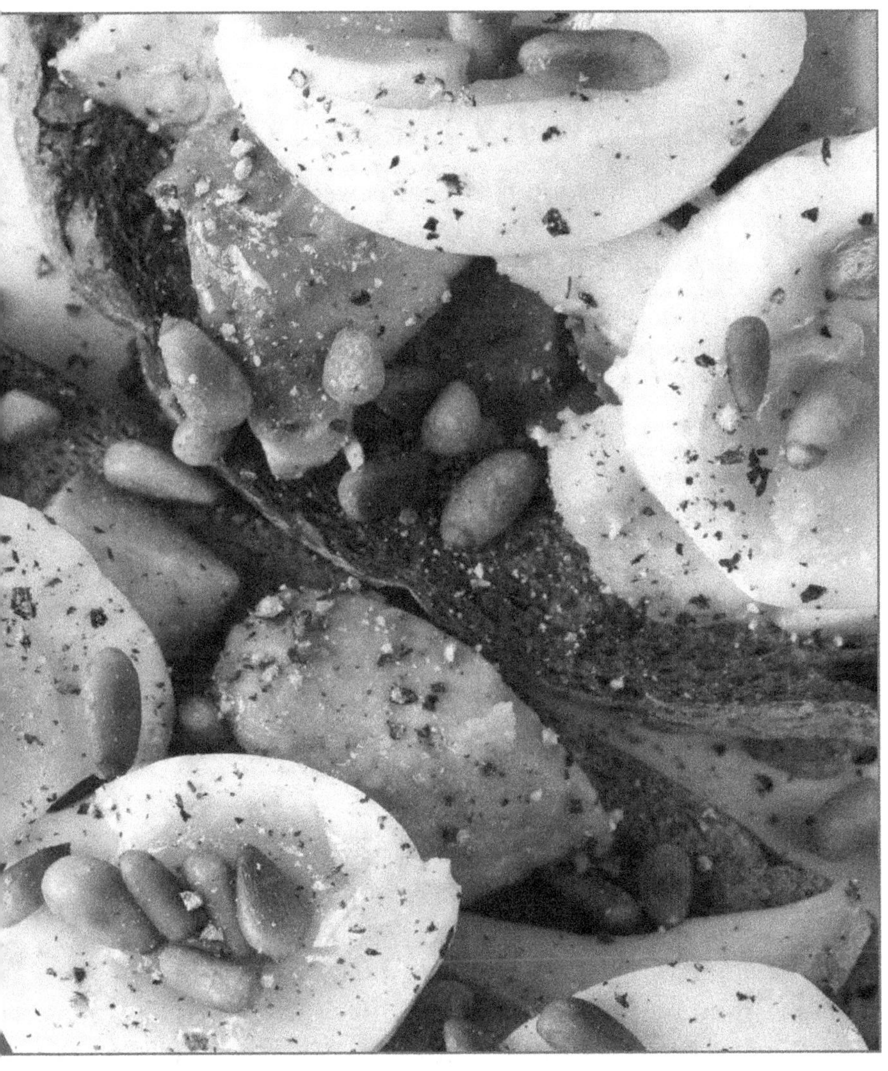

# CHAPTER 2  Meals Planning

## *2.1 The Structure of Daily Meals*

Creating a daily food plan that is well-balanced is essential to following the Carnivore Diet successfully. This entails creating a schedule that suits each person's tastes and energy requirements. A Carnivore Diet Cookbook's Daily Meal Structure section offers suggestions for distributing meals throughout the day. Some people might like to eat two large meals, while others would choose to eat three smaller ones. Including changes in the daily routine guarantees a varied intake of nutrients. The chapter places a strong emphasis on the value of paying attention to hunger signals and modifying meal schedules accordingly to promote a sustainable and sensible carnivorous lifestyle.

## *2.2 Control of Portion*

A crucial component of successfully navigating the Carnivore Diet is portion management. Knowing how to balance your consumption of fat and protein is essential in the context of this diet. The cookbook's Portion Control recommendations teach people how to adjust their serving sizes to achieve their unique nutritional objectives. It dispels the myth that a carnivorous diet calls for limitless consumption and highlights how important portion control is to overall health. The cookbook helps people achieve their ideal nutritional balance and prevents overeating by offering helpful advice and visual signals.

## 2.3 Preparing Well-Composed Meals

Meal planning for the Carnivore Diet entails more than just controlling portion sizes; it also entails combining meats with other necessary items in thoughtful ways. To guarantee a range of nutrients, practitioners are encouraged by the Cookbook's instructions on Creating Balanced Meals to include a variety of meats, organ meats, and fats. It presents the idea of nutrient density and highlights the need to obtain a complete nutritional profile at every meal. Combining various textures, flavors, and nutritional elements can help people enjoy and feel more satisfied after eating carnivorous meals. This section provides a guide for creating meals that support general health and well-being while also adhering to the principles of the Carnivore Diet.

# CHAPTER 3: Recipes for Breakfast: A Carnivorous Feast

Take a trip down the carnivorous culinary path with these breakfast dishes that are sure to make your mornings more enjoyable. Every meal, from the robust steak and eggs to the delicate salmon and cream cheese roll, is made to provide you with plenty of protein to get through the day.

## 3.1 Eggs and Steak

### Components:

8-ounce ribeye steak

Two sizable eggs

Seasoning beef with salt, pepper, and

cooked with butter or olive oil

### Getting ready:

1. Use steak seasoning, salt, and pepper to season the meat.

2. Melt butter or olive oil in a pan over medium-high heat.

3. For medium-rare, cook the steak for 3–4 minutes on each side.

4. Fry the eggs in the same skillet until the whites are set.

5. Arrange the steak and eggs on top.


***Cooking Time:*** a half hour.


### *Serving:*

Arrange the eggs and steak on a platter.

Add fresh herbs as a garnish, such as chopped chives.

Serve with grilled mushrooms for a delicious brunch.


## *3.2 Variations on Bacon and Sausage*

### ***Components:***

Six bacon slices

Four sausages of your selection

Black pepper and salt

***Preparation:***

1. Crisp up the bacon by cooking it in a frying pan.

2. Cook sausages in bacon grease till browned all over.

3. Add black pepper and salt for seasoning.

4. Present warm.

***Cooking time:*** fifteen minutes.

***Serving:***

Place the sausages and bacon on a platter.

Accompany with avocado slices or scrambled eggs.

## 3.3 Breakfast Skillet Carnivore

***Components:***

One pound of ground beef

Four eggs

Black pepper, salt, and any other flavor that you like

cooked with butter or olive oil

***Getting ready:***

1. Heat butter or olive oil in a pan to brown ground meat.

2. Crack eggs into the wells you made in the meat.

3. Cook the eggs covered until they reach your desired doneness.

4. Add desired seasoning, salt, and black pepper.

***Cooking time:*** fifteen minutes.

***Serving:***

Gently place the skillet on a serving dish.

Add chopped parsley as a garnish.

Accompany with sliced tomatoes on the side.

## 3.4 Ground beef with egg muffins

***Components:***

One pound of ground beef

Six eggs

Garlic powder, salt, and pepper

Butter or olive oil to grease the muffin pan

*Getting ready:*

1. Heat butter or olive oil in a pan to brown ground meat.

2. Beat eggs, combine with ground beef, and add garlic powder, salt, and pepper for seasoning.

3. Fill each cup of the mixture after greasing a muffin tray.

4. Bake for 12 to 15 minutes, or until eggs are set.

*Cooking time:* fifteen minutes.

*Serving Tip:*

Before serving, let the egg muffins cool somewhat.

Add some chives as a garnish and serve with avocado on the side.

3.5 Pâté of chicken liver

Components:

One pound of chicken liver

1/2 cup of butter without salt

To taste, add salt and pepper.

### Preparation

1. Clean and trim the livers of the chickens.

2. Cook livers in butter for 8 to 10 minutes, or until done.

3. Add pepper and salt for seasoning.

4. Process until smooth.

5. Store in the fridge until solid.

**Cooking Time:** a half hour.

### Serving suggestions:

Present the chicken liver paté cold.

Serve with carbohydrate-free crackers or cucumber slices.

# 3.6 Strips of pork belly

### Components:

- One pound of pork belly strips

To taste, add salt and pepper.

### Preparation

1. Set oven temperature to 400°F or 200°C.

2. Use salt and pepper to season the pork belly strips.

3. Roast for 25 to 30 minutes in the oven, or until crispy.

**Cooking Time:** half an hour.

**Serving:**

Present the hot pork belly strips.

Serve with your preferred dipping sauce or a side salad.

## 3.7 Breakfast Chops of Lamb

**Components:**

Four chops of lamb

To taste, add salt and rosemary.

**Getting ready:**

1. Use salt and rosemary to season lamb chops.

2. To taste, grill or pan-sear.

***Cooking time:*** fifteen minutes.

***Serving suggestions:***

Serve the lamb breakfast chops hot;

Serve them with sautéed spinach or scrambled eggs.

## 3.8 Cream Cheese Roll with Salmon

***Components:***

Slices of smoked salmon

Cream cheese

***Preparation:***

1. Arrange the slices of smoked salmon.

2. Cover each slice with cream cheese.

3. Form a tight log out of the salmon and cream cheese.

***Serving:***

Cut the Cream Cheese Roll and Salmon into small pieces.

Serve as a classy starter or a low-fat breakfast alternative.

The preparation process takes around ten minutes.

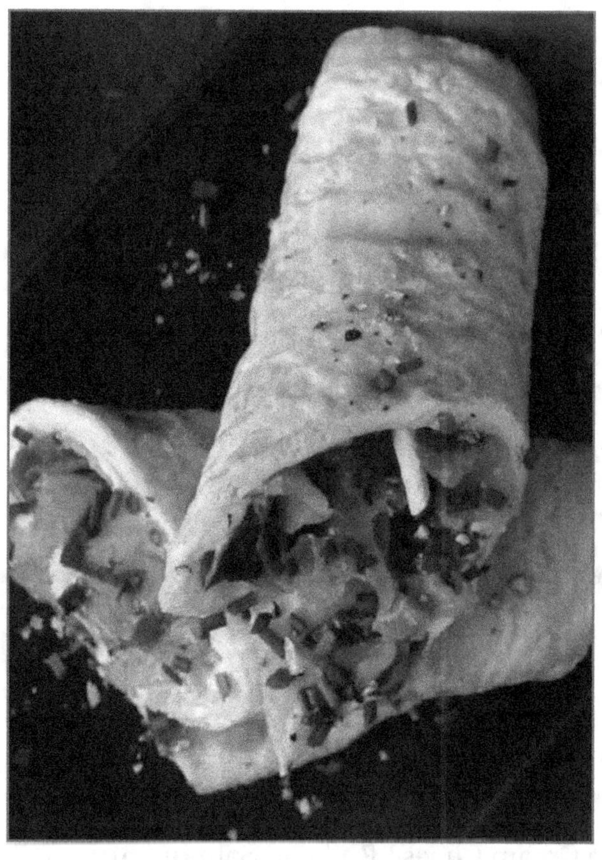

# CHAPTER 4: Lunch Ideas: A Midday Fuel Carnivore Feast

Savour a meat-filled lunch with these delectable dishes that will satisfy your noon cravings. Every item, from the filling Bison Burger Bowls to the protein-rich Grilled Chicken Salads, guarantees a tasty and healthy lunchtime.

## *4.1 Salads with Grilled Chicken*

***Components:***

Skinless and boneless chicken breasts

Assorted salad greens

Cherry tomatoes

Cucumber

Olive oil

Lemon juice

Pepper and salt

***Getting ready:***

1. Marinate chicken breasts with lemon juice, salt, pepper, and olive oil.

2. Cook the chicken completely on the grill.

3. After grilling, slice the chicken and place it over a bed of mixed leaves.

4. Add cucumber slices and cherry tomatoes as garnish.

***Cooking time:*** fifteen minutes.

***Serving:***

Garnish with a squeeze of lemon and additional olive oil.

Present as a light and high-protein salad.

## *4.2 Toppings for Beef Patties*

***Components:***

Ground beef

Leaf lettuce

Sliced tomatoes

Pickles

Mayonnaise with mustard

Pepper and salt


## Preparation

1. Add salt and pepper to the ground meat to season it.

2. Create patties out of the meat and grill them until they are done.

3. Place burgers onto leaves of lettuce.

4. Add tomato slices, pickles, mayonnaise, and mustard on top.


***Cooking Time:*** half an hour.


### Serving suggestion:

Make a meat-loving burger without the bread.

Savour with your preferred low-carb toppings.


## 4.3 Vegetables and Pork Chops

### Components:

Chops of pork

Broccoli

Bell peppers

Olive oil

Powdered garlic

Pepper and salt

**_Getting ready:_**

1. Add salt, pepper, and garlic powder to the pork chops.

2. In a heated skillet, sear the pork chops.

3. Use olive oil to roast bell peppers and broccoli.

4. Arrange roasted veggies on top of pork chops.

**_Cooking time:_** twenty minutes.

**_Serving:_**

Present the vegetables and pork chops on a platter for a filling and healthy meal.

To add even more flavor, drizzle with olive oil.

# 4.4 Wraps for Turkey Breasts

**_Components:_**

Turkey breast slices

Leaf lettuce

Slices of avocado

Strips of bacon

Mayonnaise

Pepper and salt

*Getting ready:*

1. Arrange slices of turkey on top of lettuce leaves.

2. Include cooked bacon and avocado slices.

3. Add a mayonnaise drizzle.

4. Add pepper and salt for seasoning.

*Cooking Time:*  7 minutes to fry bacon.

*Serving:*

Roll up the turkey breast wraps for an easy and delicious midday meal.

For extra crunch, serve alongside pickles.

## 4.5 Avocado and Shrimp Salad

**Components:**

Peel and deveined prawns

Diced avocado

Assorted salad greens

Lemon juice

Olive oil

Pepper and salt

**Getting ready:**

Shrimp should be sautéed in olive oil till pink.

2. Combine cooked prawns, chopped avocado, and mixed greens.

3. Drizzle with olive oil and lemon juice.

4. Add pepper and salt for seasoning.

**Cooking time:** five minutes.

**Serving:**

Serve the avocado and prawn salad as a tasty, light lunch option.

Perfect for anyone looking for a seafood-focused choice.

## 4.6 Caesar Salad for Carnivores

### Components:

Lettuce

Slices of grilled chicken

Bacon pieces

Grated Parmesan cheese

A Caesar salad

Pepper and salt

### Getting ready:

1. Arrange a platter of Romaine lettuce.

2. Add bacon pieces and slices of cooked chicken on top.

3. Add grated Parmesan cheese on top.

4. Add a Caesar dressing drizzle.

### Serving:

Present the Carnivore Caesar Salad as a filling and substantial midday meal.

A classic with a meat-loving sensibility.

## 4.7 Bowls of Bison Burgers

**Components:**

Bison on the ground

Rice made from cauliflower

Slices of avocado

A finely sliced red onion

Mayonnaise with mustard

Pepper and salt

**Getting ready:**

1. Sprinkle salt and pepper over the ground bison.

2. Shape into patties and fry till desired.

3. Put on top of cauliflower rice.

4. Add red onion and avocado slices on top.

5. Drizzle with mayonnaise and mustard.

***Cooking time:*** fifteen minutes.

***Serving:***

Savour the low-carb and filling Bison Burger Bowls for lunch.

Tight with flavor and protein.

## *4.8 Lettuce Wraps with Tuna Salad*

***Components:***

Drain and can tuna

Finely sliced celery

Diced red bell pepper

Mayonnaise

Mustard dijon

Leaf lettuce

Pepper and salt

***Getting ready:***

Combine the tuna, red bell pepper, celery, mayonnaise, and Dijon mustard in a bowl.

2. Add pepper and salt for seasoning.

3. Spoon the lettuce leaves with the tuna mixture.

4. Tie with toothpicks and wrap.

### *Serving:*

Present Tuna Salad Lettuce Wraps as a filling and light lunch choice.

Ideal for anybody in the mood for something light and high in protein.

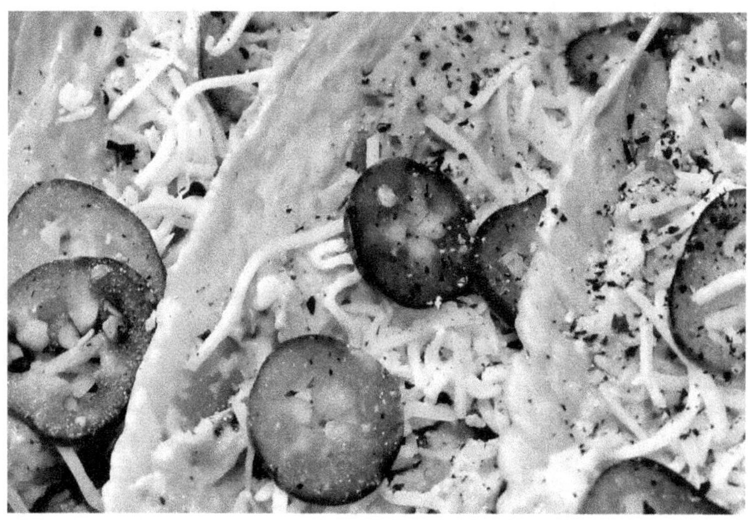

# CHAPTER 5: Dinner Treats: Carnivorous Elegance for After-hours Pleasure

Savor the elegance of carnivorous richness with our Dinner Delights. Every recipe, from the delicious Duck Breast with Orange Glaze to the juicy Lamb Chops with Herbs, is a symphony of flavors that are expertly prepared to enrich your dining experience. Let your inner carnivore go and enjoy these delicious recipes.

## 5.1 Herb-Crusted Lamb Chops

### Components:

Four chops of lamb

Fresh thyme and rosemary

Cloves of garlic

Black pepper and salt

Olive oil

***Getting ready:***

1. Season lamb chops with chopped herbs, salt, and pepper.

2. Mash the garlic and rub it across the chops.

3. Sear till golden in olive oil.

4. Bake the food until it's done.

***Cooking time:*** twenty minutes.

***Serving:***

Add more herbs as garnish.

Accompany with roasted veggie side dishes.

## 5.2 Butter-Poached Ribeye Steak

***Components:***

A pair of ribeye steaks

Black pepper and salt

Butter

Cloves of garlic

New thyme

***Getting ready:***

1. Use salt and pepper to season the steaks.

2. Sear with butter, garlic, and thyme in a heated skillet.

3. Cook till the doneness you desire.

***Cooking time:*** fifteen minutes.

***Serving:***

Apply a butter-melted glaze.

Accompany with a serving of velvety mashed cauliflower.

## 5.3 Seafood and Fish Fillets

***Components:***

A variety of fish fillets

Scallops with prawns

Lemon juice and zest

Olive oil

New parsley

Pepper and salt

***Getting ready:***

1. Use lemon zest, salt, and pepper to season fish fillets and seafood.

2. Sear till cooked through in olive oil.

3. Add a lemon juice drizzle and parsley garnish.

***Cooking Time:*** half an hour.

***Serving:***

Arrange on top of some sautéed spinach.

Savour with a squeeze of lemon, fresh.

## 5.4 Rosemary Chicken Thighs

***Components:***

Chicken tenders

Newly harvested rosemary

Powdered garlic

Black pepper and salt

Olive oil

***Getting ready:***

1. Season chicken thighs with garlic powder, salt, and pepper.

2. Add a dash of recently harvested rosemary.

3. Bake until well done and golden.

***Cooking Time:***  half an hour.

***Serving:***

As a garnish, add more rosemary.

Serve with roasted Brussels sprouts for dipping.

# *5.5 Stuffed Bell Peppers with Ground Beef*

***Components:***

Bell peppers

Ground beef

Garlic with onions

Sauce made from tomatoes

Seasoning from Italy

Black pepper and salt


***Getting ready:***

1. Add the ground beef and sauté it with the onion and garlic until it browns.

2. Stir in spice and tomato sauce.

3. After stuffing bell peppers, bake them until they are soft.


***Cooking Time:*** twenty-five minutes.


***Serving:***

Sprinkle grated cheese on top.

Accompany by a side salad.


## 5.6 Dry-Rub Pork Ribs

***Components:***

Ribs of pork

Cayenne, paprika, and garlic powder

Brown sugar, if used

Black pepper and salt

***Getting ready:***

1. Apply a dry rub to the ribs using paprika, cayenne, garlic powder, salt, and pepper.

2. Bake or grill until soft.

***Cooking Time:*** two hours.

***Serving:***

Drizzle with a barbecue sauce with smoke.

Accompany with coleslaw.

## 5.7 Mushroom-Crusted Venison Steaks

***Components:***

Steaks of venison

Mushrooms

Red wine

Cloves of garlic

Thyme

Black pepper and salt


***Getting ready:***

1. Sear steaks of venison to a medium-rare color.

2. Saute the garlic, thyme, and mushrooms.

3. Use red wine to deglaze.


***Cooking time:*** fifteen minutes.


***Serving:***

Sprinkle the venison with mushrooms.

Accompany with mashed cauliflower flavored with garlic.


## 5.8 Glazed Duck Breast in Orange

***Components:***

Duck breasts

Zest and orange juice

Honey

Soy sauce

Ginger

Black pepper and salt

***Getting ready:***

1. Score the skin of the duck and season with pepper and salt.

Sear until the skin becomes crispy.

3. Use a glaze made of ginger, soy sauce, orange juice, zest, and honey.

***Cooking time:*** twenty minutes.

***Serving:***

Cut the duck into slices and pour orange glaze over it.

Accompany with steaming asparagus.

# CHAPTER 6: Carnivore Temptations: Snacks & Quick Bites for Any Time

Savour delicious treats from our assortment of snacks and quick bites, which are ideal for sating your appetite in between meals. Every snack, from the delicious Smoked Salmon Rolls to the tempting Parmesan Crisps, is painstakingly made for both taste and ease of use. These recipes have been certified by carnivores, so step up your snack game.

## 6.1 Jerky Beef

***Components:***

Strips of beef

Soy sauce

Worcestershire sauce

Powdered garlic

Powdered onion

Pepper, black

***Preparation:***

1. Start by marinating beef strips in a concoction of Worcestershire sauce, soy sauce, onion powder, garlic powder, and black pepper.

2. Bake or dehydrate the jerky until it becomes delicious and dry.

***Cooking Period:***

Dehydration: four to six hours.

Baking time: around four hours.

***Serving:***

Savour the protein-rich and portable Beef Jerky snack.

## *6.2 Rolls with Cheese*

***Components:***

Cheese slices, either mozzarella or cheddar

Slices of pepperoni or salami

***Getting ready:***

1. Arrange cheese slices on top of salami or pepperoni pieces.

2. Tightly roll up.


**Serving:**

Present the cheese rolls as a filling and speedy low-carbohydrate snack.


## 6.3 Eggs Hard-Boiled

**Components:**

Eggs


**Getting ready:**

1. Boiled eggs until set in the yolks.


Cooking time is around ten to twelve minutes.


**Serving suggestions:**

 For a traditional and practical snack, season with salt and pepper.

## 6.4 Cream Cheese and Salami Bites

**Components:**

Slices of salami

Cream cheese

**Getting ready:**

1. Spread slices of salami with cream cheese.

2. Tightly roll up.

**Serving suggestion:**

Savor these delicious bite-sized morsels of salami and cream cheese for a fast and savory snack.

## 6.5 Lemon-Crusted Sardines

**Components:**

Sardines in cans

Slicing lemons

**Getting ready:**

1. Open the sardines can.

2. Drizzle the sardines with lemon juice.

***Serving suggestion:***

Savour the Sardines with Lemon as a nutrient-dense, zesty snack.

## 6.6 Eggs deviled with bacon

***Components:***

Hard-boiled eggs

Mayonnaise

Mustard

Bacon pieces

Paprika

***Getting ready:***

1. Halve the hard-boiled eggs.

2. Combine bacon pieces, mustard, and mayonnaise with yolks.

3. Fill egg halves with mixture using a spoon.

4. Add paprika to the mixture.

**Serving suggestions:**

As a tasty snack, savor the creamy and savory Deviled Eggs with Bacon.


# 6.7 Rolls with Smoked Salmon

**Components:**

Slices of smoked salmon

Cream cheese

Chives


**Getting ready:**

1. Drizzle smoked salmon pieces with cream cheese.

2. Tightly roll up.

3. Add chopped chives as a garnish.


**Serving:**

Savor the sophistication of Smoked Salmon Rolls as a chic little snack.

# 6.8 Crisps with Parmesan Cheese

## Components:

Cheese Parmesan, grated

## Getting ready:

1. On a baking sheet, shape little mounds of Parmesan cheese.

2. Bake until crisp and brown.

**Cooking time:** five to seven minutes.

## Serving:

Snackle up on these crispy Parmesan Crisps for a filling and ketogenic snack.

With these fast and simple carnivore nibbles, you can up your snack game and make sure that your desires are satisfied with satisfying, healthy alternatives all day long.

# CONCLUSION

By the time this carnivorous adventure concludes, it will be evident that this book is about more than just recipes and meal planning. It honors the ancestors' bond with the bountiful food supply of the animal kingdom and humankind. As these pages explore, the carnivorous lifestyle is more than simply a diet; it's a way of thinking that celebrates health, simplicity, and giving in to our primal desires.

In the kitchen, we've mastered the technique of turning premium meats into a flavorful symphony, from the delicate richness of organ meats to the perfectly seared perfection of steak. The Sample Meal Plans offer a methodical yet adaptable strategy that leads novices and experienced meat eaters alike through a wide range of foods that enhance the dining experience.

Recipes are just one part of the process; there is also learning about the carnivorous attitude, meal planning, and adopting sophisticated tactics. This book is an extensive manual that will enable you to tailor your carnivorous odyssey to your tastes and objectives.

As you relish the last pages, may you go move out on your carnivorous journey with assurance, equipped with the understanding to fuel your physique and satisfy your taste buds? May the carnivorous lifestyle become a sustainable and satisfying aspect of your culinary identity, and may every meal serve as a reminder of the inherent delight found in simplicity. Raise a glass to a life well-lived via the path of the carnivore and its primitive joys!

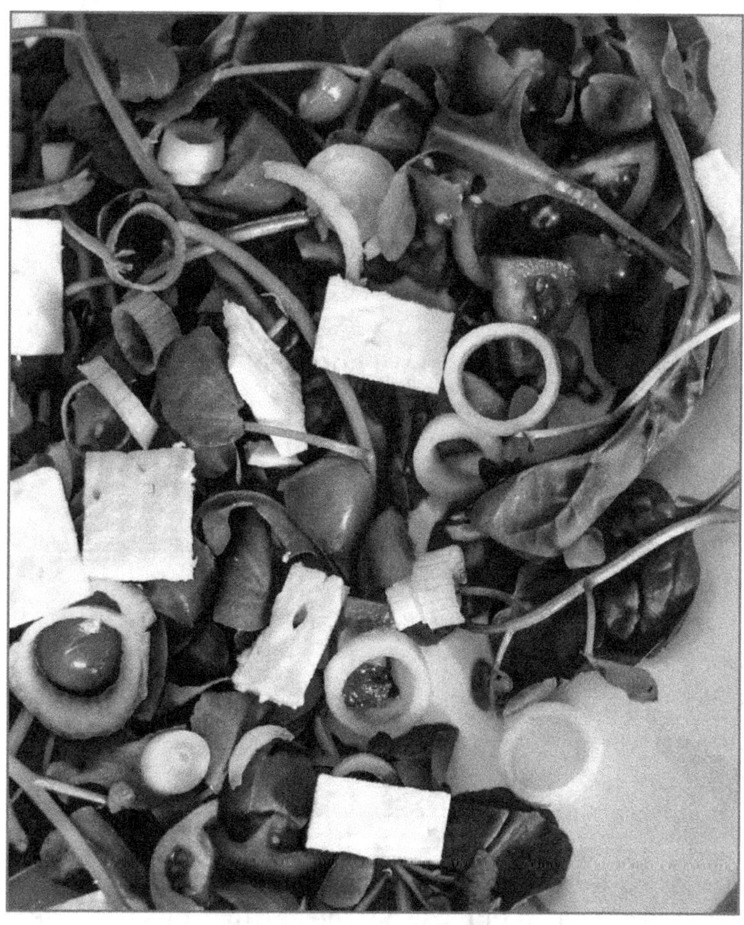

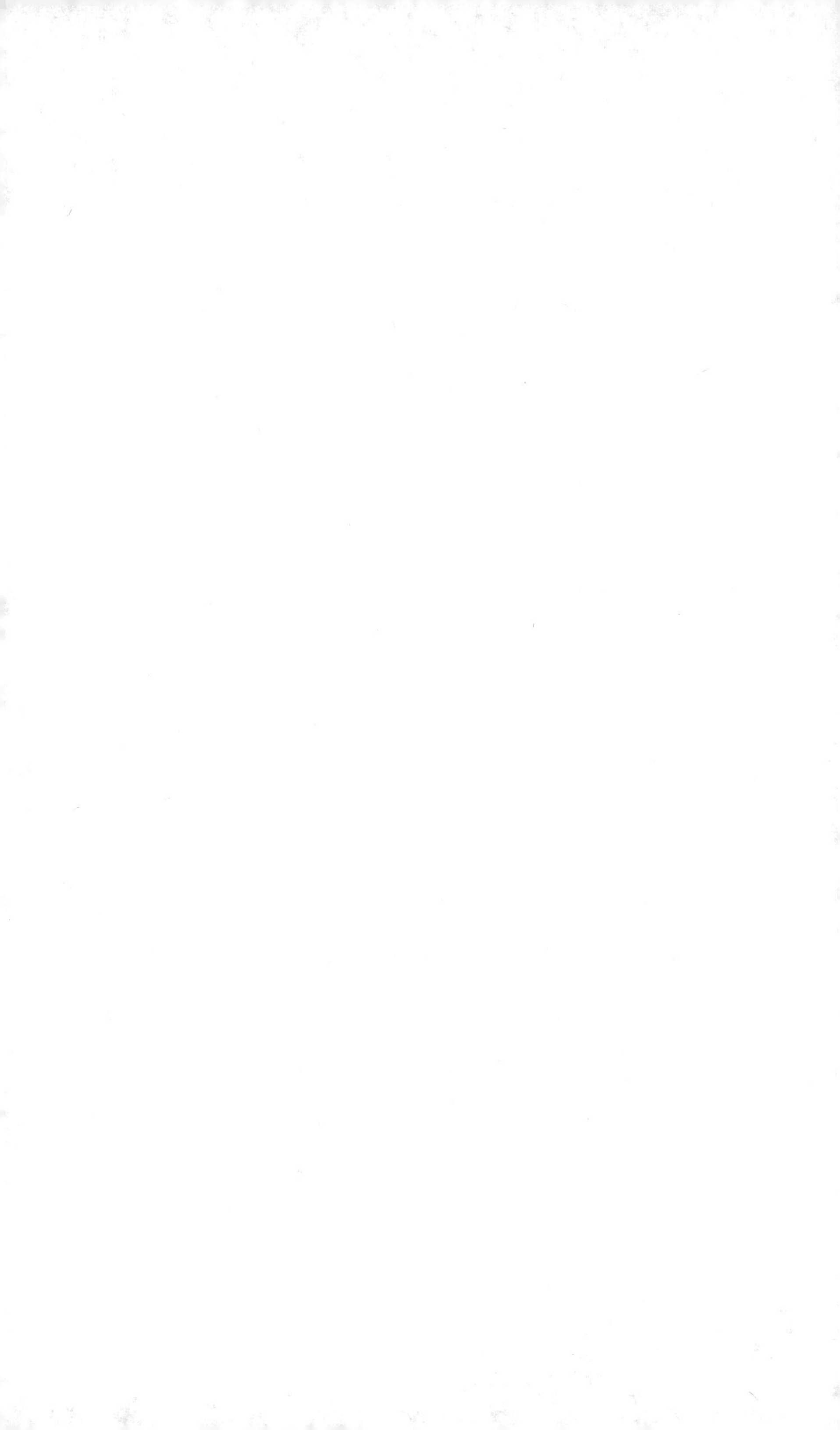

www.ingramcontent.com/pod-product-compliance
Lightning Source LLC
Chambersburg PA
CBHW070734260726
48660CB00007B/2845